Lyn Marshall's
KEEP UP WITH
YOGA

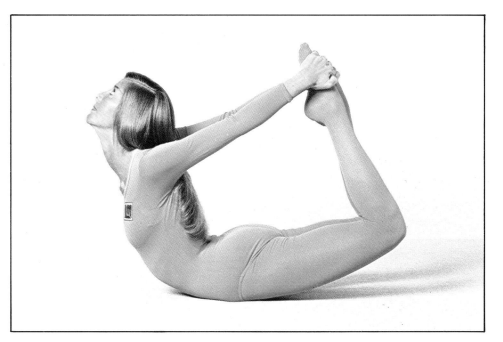

The reining in of the body
The tranquillity of the mind
The sensation of slightly floating
As one lets oneself unwind

The feeling of unification
With body and soul as one
Great peace and inner contentment
For you know – it has only begun.

L. M.

WARD LOCK LIMITED·LONDON

© Yoga World Limited 1976

ISBN 0 7063 5236 X

First published in 1976 in Great Britain by
Ward Lock Limited, 82 Gower Street,
London WC1E 6EQ, a Pentos Company.

Second Impression 1977
Third Impression 1978
Fourth Impression 1981
Fifth Impression 1982

Photographs by Simon Farrell

Printed and bound in Singapore by
Kyodo-Shing Loong Printing Industries Pte Ltd.

Contents

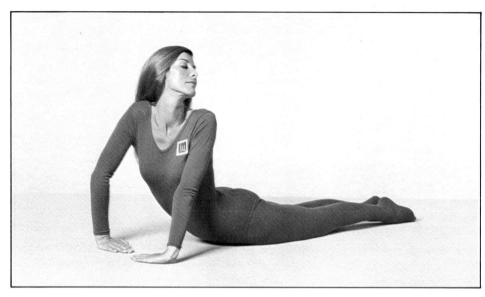

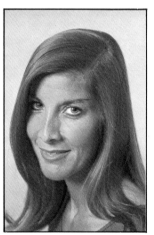

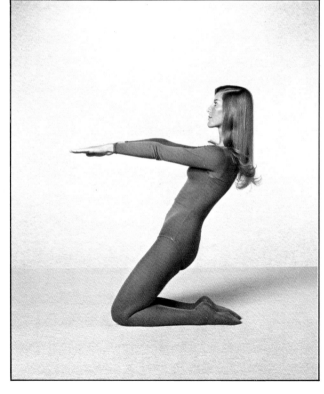

Introduction

If you have just purchased this book and are new to Yoga, I would like to welcome you as one of my new students, and to tell you that you are on your way to discovering the most PERFECT and NATURAL form of physical and mental improvement ever devised by man.

You will see in the subsequent pages that Yoga done my way is effortless and extremely enjoyable. What's more, you will feel its benefits as soon as you begin to practise.

You need spend only a few minutes a day practising to receive the tremendous rewards that Yoga can bring.

I am thrilled at the vast number of people now practising my method of Yoga, and I hope that you too will join them and that your life will be greatly enriched by your Yoga practice. I would like to wish you every success with your practice, and to express my joy in the knowledge that now through my books, television programmes and records, I am able to reach so many people and share the thing that I value most in life – my Yoga teaching.

Lyn Marshall

Please Note

The illustrations and instructions for each movement are very clearly set out and easy to follow, but before you begin to practise it is important that you understand a little about my style of Yoga, so please read the following pages carefully.

Although it is perfectly all right for you to begin practising with this book, I would recommend that you also get a copy of *Wake up to Yoga* as it includes many other elementary postures and positions that will help prepare you for some of the more advanced positions shown in this book.

What is Yoga?

Physical or Hatha Yoga is a series of extremely well thought out postures or positions that move and improve virtually every part of the human body.

They are not exercizes, but if you practise the Yoga movements regularly, it is easy to reach peak physical condition, spending very little time and a minimum of effort. This is quite the reverse of the normal rigorous activities that one expects to have to undertake to improve one's body and health.

There are many self-improvement gadgets on the market as well as numerous services, all claiming that they will DO IT FOR YOU. Well, although some of these might work for a period of time, the effect can only be temporary. Permanent body improvement must come from inside your own body. It must be a natural body movement, and Yoga done my way is not only natural and enjoyable, but its effectiveness can be felt as soon as you start to practise.

In short—it works.

My Method

My method of Yoga is first and foremost very pleasurable to do. It is not a physical workout of any sort, but a series of gentle stretches that when put together become the Yoga movements.

There are various forms of physical or Hatha Yoga being practised today. Many of them place great emphasis on attaining the finished positions or postures, and this has unfortunately caused many would-be students to drop out. They find it either too much of a strain to get into these positions, or, as many are unable to get anywhere near to achieving the positions, they feel that continuing would be totally pointless.

With my method of Yoga, there is no finished position that one **has** to attain. Emphasis is placed on moving slowly and smoothly, and the amount of stretching that you do to begin with is so slight as to be hardly noticeable. You stop as soon as you reach your own body's natural and comfortable limit, and it is by holding this position still for a set count that you establish the stretch in the body and limbs. Each time you come to repeat the movement you are then able to go a little further.

The Importance of Moving Slowly

Moving slowly is very important, because if you move slowly you are aware of your body and can feel exactly when you have gone far enough – and you stop. Moving quickly, you know you have gone too far only when it is too late, and the muscles or ligaments are pulled and the damage is done. Also, by moving slowly, you are able to concentrate completely on the particular section of the body that is being exercized, and this automatically clears the mind of all other thoughts. This clearance of the mind, even if it is only for a few short minutes, brings about tremendous mental relaxation.

You may find that moving slowly is a little difficult at first because we are so used to doing everything quickly, but as you practise and become more aware of your body, you will find yourself slowing down.

Competition

There is no such thing as competition in Yoga. Every **body** is different, and it does not matter that one person can get into a seemingly advanced position in a week of practice while another is still in a comparatively elementary position after practising for nearly a year. As long as you go to your own comfortable limit, you will be getting the same amount of benefit no matter what stage of the position you are in. Likewise, it does not follow that someone who is slim and athletic will progress any faster than a middle-aged person who is of heavy build. So be aware only of yourself. There is no hurry and no prize for the person who reaches a certain position first. You will be receiving full benefit from your first day of practice, because you are listening to your body and allowing it to take you a little further only when it is ready.

Not Straining

It is important that you never ever strain or try to go further than your body will allow in any of the positions. Trying to do too much too quickly will only retard your progress not accelerate it. We are so used to putting in a lot of effort when exercizing our bodies, that you may find it a little difficult at first actually to stop yourself from going that little bit further. A phrase that I have often heard used when people refer to physical exercize is **'it has to hurt to do you good'**. Well, this certainly is not true of Yoga. Your Yoga practice should be one of the most enjoyable parts of your day.

Names of Movements

All of my movements and postures have easily identifiable English names, and as you practise, these will quickly become familiar to you.

The Value of Yoga

The value of my style of Yoga is that it is designed for people who lead normal lives, and whether you are young or old, fat or thin, you can fit it into your life and use it in a practical way to achieve any or all of the following:

Lose weight – either generally or in specific areas of the body.
Learn how to relax properly.
Rid yourself of back problems.
Remove mental strain and tension.
Improve your figure.
Strengthen and recondition your entire body.
Stay relaxed under pressure.
Improve your concentration.
Become more sensually aware of yourself and others.
Improve your circulation and breathing.
Get relief from conditions such as insomnia, headache, migraine, sinusitis and asthma.
Improve the condition of your skin, your eyes and your hair.
Improve your balance and posture.
Eliminate feelings of depression.
Regain agility and youth.

Yes, you can use the movements for all of these things and many many more, far too numerous to mention.

You may feel that this claim seems somewhat exaggerated, and I would urge you to practise the movements–the results will be all the proof you need.

I believe that one Yoga movement executed **my way** is of more value than ten normal exercizes, and for this reason seldom is any movement performed more than twice. The normal repetitive 1–2, 1–2 type exercizes can not only become monotonous, but they also tend to overactivate the heart, putting a strain on it, to increase the appetite, to cause perspiration and a feeling of exhaustion – and usually relief when it is all over.

My Yoga movements, on the other hand, leave you feeling refreshed, relaxed, invigorated and revitalized – even if you spend just a few minutes doing them.

Practice

Practise any of the movements whenever you have the time and space, preferably somewhere quiet where you won't be disturbed. You can do just one or as many of the postures as you wish. To begin with, however, I suggest that you do not set yourself a rigid practice routine that you force yourself to go through every day. Spend just a few minutes performing one or maybe two of the movements that you really enjoy. Then, as time goes by, like most things in life that you enjoy, you will find yourself wanting to spend more and more time practising.

When you want to start practising a series of movements in the form of a session, never try to do as many movements as you can. You will probably rush them and get very little benefit. Slowness and smoothness is the key, and it is far better to spend ten minutes doing one movement correctly than four or five hurriedly.

Practise with as little food in the stomach as possible (preferably no food for at least an hour and a half before your session).

The movements you choose for your session are up to you, but try to get a good balance by doing movements that will get to all parts of the body. I have worked out some Practice Routines for twenty and thirty minutes on page 77 and you might like to try these.

It is very important to relax in the Corpse position (the posture of deep relaxation) for a few minutes both at the beginning and at the end of your session, and also to relax, as instructed, after each movement.

Many people now practise Yoga while at work during the day, often taking a portion of their lunch break, and this is fine. If you have colleagues or workmates who are also interested in practising, then why not organize a group practice session? Remember to eat after your session though – not before.

Ideally, the room that you practise in should be well ventilated, allowing as much fresh air into the room as possible. In the summer, of course, it is perfectly all right to practise out of doors.

Practice Clothes

You should be able to move your body quite freely, without anything tight or restricting around the waist. The most practical clothes are a leotard and tights for women, and trousers or shorts with an elasticated waistband for men. If you are going to practise the movements at work and find it impossible to change, loosen your clothing around the waist and take your shoes off.

Yoga Practice Mats

Floor surfaces do vary a great deal, and if you are going to practise regularly then it is well worth investing in a Yoga practice mat. These are specially designed so that they are not only firm enough to support you and allow you to balance properly, but have sufficient give to cushion the bones and joints in some of the sitting, kneeling and lying postures. These mats can be packed away and kept clean between your practice sessions, and can be used indoors or out.

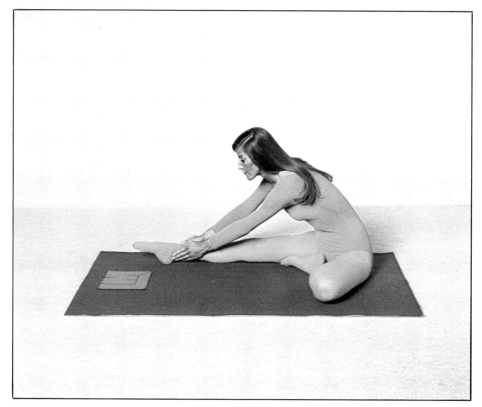

Yoga and Children

Children take very easily to this form of movement and enjoy it tremendously. As well as receiving the physical benefits of Yoga, I believe that it gives them a sense of body awareness that they do not get from the sports and P.E. generally taught in schools. Also, there is no element of competition in Yoga, and this often helps to remove any feelings of inadequacy that a child may develop if he is not able to perform the physical activities taught in school as well as his contemporaries.

Never pressure your child to do Yoga, he will regard it as work and resent it. If you practise, you will probably find that your child's natural inquisitiveness will lead him to ask what you are doing and he will want to join in. Encourage this and allow him to practise with you. Then, when you are sure the child knows the movements, and is old enough, he or she can practise alone if preferred. Children vary considerably, and you must judge for yourself at what age your child is responsible enough to practise the movements unsupervised.

Children's limbs are extremely supple, and it is up to you to restrain them from attempting any of the advanced positions shown. Although they may be able to get into these positions quite easily, it could do them harm. So ensure that they stick to the simple movements and modified positions only.

As children grow older, Yoga practice will help them in their studies by improving their concentration and mental alertness. They will also be calmer in situations where stress and tension often prevail, like exam time.

Once a child learns the movements and postures, the probability is that he will continue to practise them throughout his entire life.

Note

I would recommend that a child does not begin to practise until the age of five or six.

If your child is unwell, or has a medical condition – you must get your doctor's approval before allowing your child to start to practise. The same applies if your child has a history of either mental or physical illness.

Yoga and Senior Citizens

Many people have said 'Am I too old to begin practising' Yoga?', and the answer is a very definite NO. People of all ages can begin to practise Yoga, and there is no reason why you should not start at sixty, seventy or even eighty years of age.

The important thing to remember is that you do not have to go very far in order to get results and benefits. The movements are progressive, and no matter how stiff or out of condition you are to begin with, if you execute the movements gently and carefully – never straining – you will find yourself able to go further and further as your body stretches naturally.

It has been my experience that Yoga movements can be particularly beneficial where chronic stiffening of the joints has occurred, as in osteo-arthritis, and a great degree of success can be achieved with patient, regular and gentle practice of the movements. However, if you are suffering from this or any other medical condition, DO consult your doctor before commencing with your practice.

Yoga and Sex

It is not surprising that the practice of Yoga brings about a marked improvement in your sex life.

To begin with, your ability to relax is greatly increased, and the smooth, gentle and unhurried way in which the movements are performed will bring about an acute feeling of body awareness. You will begin to revel in the enjoyment that moving your body in this way brings, and you will derive a positive sensual pleasure when doing the movements. This feeling of pleasure in moving your own body will wash over into your normal everyday activities, and you will find yourself becoming more aware of how you walk, sit, stand and move generally. This sensual pleasure can be enjoyed to its fullest extent when making love.

You will find that your ability both to give and to receive physical love and affection increases as time goes by, and you will experience a great heightening of the senses such as touch, taste, smell and feel, all of which will greatly contribute to the enjoyment of love making.

A good and satisfying sexual relationship can only be achieved through mental as well as physical communication, and through the practice of Yoga your inhibitions will go and your natural desire to touch and be touched can be expressed freely. Your sensitivity toward your partner increases, so that you are able to understand his or her needs and desires also.

A slightly more practical reason why your sex life will improve is the fact that you are toning up and strengthening areas of the body that are particularly relevant during love making, and your body is therefore better equipped to perform the act of intercourse. Your glands too are being made to function efficiently, which has a very positive effect on your sex life.

Over the years, many students of all ages have told me how much their physical relationships have improved. Some have been very surprised that the practice of the Yoga movements could do this, but without exception all have been delighted.

Yoga and Pregnancy

There is no reason why you should not practise Yoga when you are pregnant. As well as keeping your body supple and strong, it will also help prepare your body for the actual birth, and promote the speedy recovery of your figure after the baby is born. Obviously great care must be taken with the choice of movements, so as not to undertake anything that could be dangerous either to you or to your unborn child.

Subject to your doctor's prior approval, you can practise the movements recommended in the Ante-Natal section of the book. You will find as your pregnancy continues that you are less prone to fatigue, and not inclined to put on unnecessary weight, as is common in pregnancy. You will also learn the art of deep breathing and relaxation, which will be an invaluable asset during the actual birth, and you will develop a general feeling of extreme well-being.

The period immediately after your baby is born is crucial, and the muscles should be made to work again as quickly as possible. This is vital if you are to prevent sagging, and no matter how small the effort is to begin with – it must be made. Many women tell me that the post-natal depression that often accompanies childbirth has not been experienced when they have been practising the Yoga movements. This, I think, can be partially attributed to the fact that if a woman can see her figure returning quickly she is not likely to be depressed over her appearance – she will be delighted by it and by the continued improvement that follows.

There are actually movements that you can do as soon as the day after your baby is born, just lying or sitting up in bed, and although these movements are very subtle they really are very effective. However, before you commence these, or any other movements, you must obtain the full permission of your doctor.

You will find the Ante- and Post-Natal section on pages 55 to 69.

Does Yoga Change Your Life?

You do not have to alter your life one bit to practise Yoga, but changes will occur. The first and most obvious change is that you will both look and feel better. Also, the more you practise, the more you will find subtle little changes taking place. For example, you tend to slow down and relax more when eating, and many people tell me that they suddenly realize that they are satisfied with far less food than they were previously used to.

Sensitivity and awareness increase, and you may find that your taste buds become more alive and you go off certain foods, developing preferences for others. This is not something that you make yourself do, it just seems to happen over a period of time. Likewise, a lot of students tell me that they have cut down on their smoking without consciously setting out to do so. The nice thing about these changes is that invariably they are for the better. Who, after all, wants to continue to smoke heavily with the threat of lung cancer hanging over them? Moreover, there is never a feeling of deprivation, since you do not set out to bring about these changes – they just happen naturally.

You may also find that your approach to life changes, as tension, worry and anxiety gradually disappear. These negative and energy-wasting elements will be replaced by a much more positive attitude to life.

It is a pity, but also understandable, that so many people today are existing in a constant state of high tension, thinking and worrying about tomorrow. But what about today? Today is LIFE—enjoy it now before it is gone for ever. That doesn't mean to say that you should opt out of your responsibilities. It simply means that with the removal of tension, worry and anxiety, you are much better equipped to deal with your normal day-to-day problems calmly and efficiently—AND—to experience the pure joy of living right HERE and right NOW, every minute of every day.

Through the practice of Yoga you will come to realize that you are your own true master, and if you do not wish to become tense or anxious, you will not allow yourself to become so. It is that simple.

Yoga and Breathing

A lot of people become very worried when Yoga breathing is mentioned. They think it is a complex technique that is very difficult to understand and practise. It is not – it is natural and you are probably breathing correctly right now. Yoga breathing is done from the abdomen rather than the chest, and this simply means that when a deep breath is taken it is taken lower down, allowing the abdomen to expand first as it fills with breath, then the diaphragm and finally the chest. The most marked difference between this and the way we normally take a deep breath is that we tend to expand the chest only, and by comparison this is a shallow breath taking in much less air and oxygen.

I do not want you to become preoccupied with the breathing to begin with, as this will only result in confusion. Simply learn the movements thoroughly, breathing normally and slowly through the nose. Then, when you have become quite proficient in the movements, start to follow the breathing instructions. At first you will probably find yourself taking the breath in the familiar way – expanding the chest only – and this is perfectly all right. You may also find at first that you cannot hold the breath for the recommended count, as instructed. Do not worry. This, like everything else, takes a little practice, so either come out of the position or simply take another breath. You will find that with time you are able to retain the breath for longer and longer periods quite comfortably.

When the time arrives, and you want to start practising abdominal breathing, I think you will find the exercize which is shown on page 22 of great value.

Medical Cautions

Though it is clear that Yoga improves your health and can also be very therapeutic in eliminating many physical ailments and disorders, **it must never ever be used as a substitute for medical treatment.**

If you are suffering from ANY condition, no matter how mild, or have a history of illness, **then you must check with your doctor before you begin to practise.** He knows your medical history and is therefore qualified to tell you whether you can safely undertake these movements.

If your doctor is not familiar with this method of Yoga, show him this book and explain the manner in which the movements are performed – slowly and smoothly. He may feel that certain of the movements may be beneficial to you whilst others should be avoided, so take care to follow his advice.

Many doctors are now realizing the benefits and advantages that Yoga done this way has to offer, and as well as having many doctors among my students, I am finding that more and more doctors are referring patients to me. The extreme gentleness of this form of Yoga often makes it the ideal system of body movement for patients who must not or who cannot undertake strenuous exercize.

Points to Remember

1 Although the Yoga movements are both easy and pleasurable to do, you must approach them in a serious manner if you are to get maximum benefit out of them.

2 Whether you practise for three or thirty minutes, devote all your attention to what you are doing and try to concentrate completely on whichever part of the body is being used.

3 The holding count for most of the positions is five. Count to yourself at approximately the same speed as seconds. Where the count differs, you will find it clearly indicated in my instructions.

4 Remember to do **everything** slowly and smoothly. This rule applies not only while doing the actual postures, but also when you lie down or get up before and after a movement. Don't rush—do it slowly.

5 As well as executing the movements and postures correctly, it is also very important to allow your body to unwind at its own natural pace after performing a movement. So, whether you are continuing with another movement or returning to the day's activities, take care to spend at least a few moments in the relaxation positions as shown, following certain movements.

6 Read the instructions relating to each movement or posture and study the pictures carefully before you attempt to perform it.

7 Great care should be taken to position the body exactly as directed, and even though the placement of fingers, elbows, chin etc. may seem trivial, they are of infinite importance to the movements.

8 It is important to relax in the Corpse position (the posture of deep relaxation) as shown on page 20 both at the beginning and at the end of your practice session for at least a few minutes.

The Movements

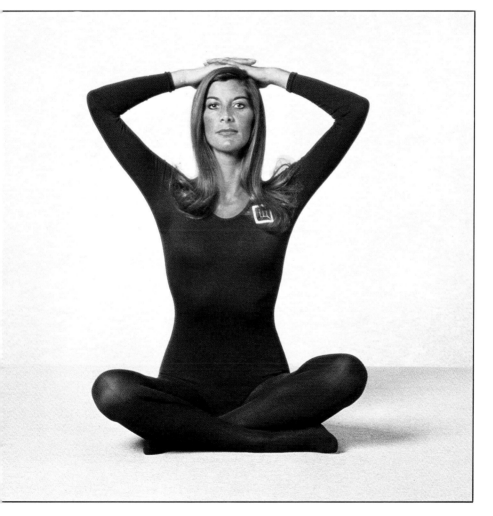

The Corpse

The Corpse, or posture of deep relaxation, must always be adopted for a few minutes both before and after your Yoga session. It should also be used to relax the body completely before and after any of the movements that are done lying on the back.

The Corpse posture when used on its own is extremely effective in refreshing, relaxing and revitalizing the entire body. Maintain the position for as long as your time allows.

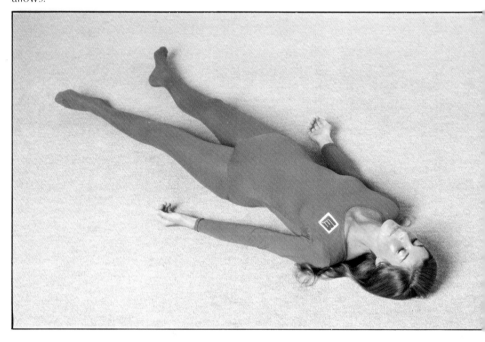

Note the way the legs and feet are positioned to allow total relaxation. The same applies to the arms and hands. Always close the eyes when relaxing like this.

Relaxation on Stomach

This position should always be adopted both before and after executing any movements that are done lying on the stomach.

The face is placed on the cheek. The heels are allowed to fall right open relaxing the legs and feet completely, and the elbows are slightly bent to relax the shoulders, arms and hands.

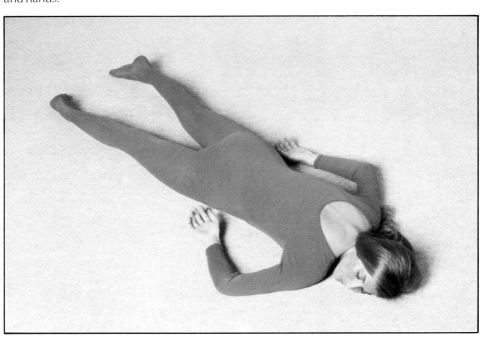

Abdominal Breathing

By practising this breathing exercize a few times each day, you will find that abdominal breathing eventually becomes quite natural, and you can then incorporate it into your Yoga practice.

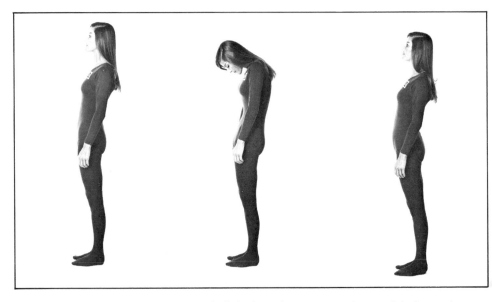

1 Stand with the back straight and your arms loosely relaxed at your sides.

2 Expel all the breath in the body by contracting the abdomen as you exhale through the nose, letting the head and shoulders relax forward a little.

3 Start to inhale gently, allowing the abdomen to expand first, then the diaphragm and finally the chest.

Hold the breath for a few seconds and then exhale slowly, reversing the process. So the chest will sink down and contract, followed by the diaphragm and the abdomen, and let the head and shoulders relax over once more.

Repeat the movement as many times as you wish.

Initially, you can help yourself to achieve the correct movement by pushing the abdomen out slightly as you inhale, and contracting it as you expel the air.

Standing Slide Bend

This is a nice gentle movement that will reduce excess weight from the waist, as well as stretching the sides of the body and eliminating stiffness from the neck. It will also improve your sense of balance.

To begin with do not try to slide your hand down to the knee as shown in picture 2. Bend as far as is comfortable. In time, as your sides stretch, you will be able to bend further and further over.

You must remember to move slowly and smoothly all the time while executing this movement.

Breathing
Inhale deeply through the nose when upright – hold the breath as you bend to the side – exhale slowly during the count – inhale as you straighten up – and exhale as the head relaxes forward, ready to repeat on other side.

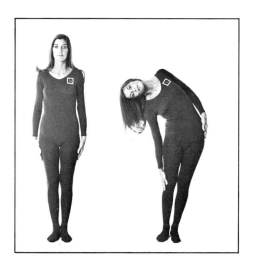

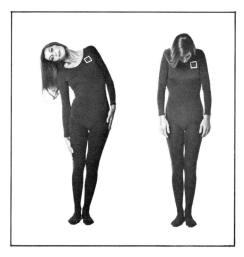

1 Stand straight with the legs and feet together and the head erect. Place the palms of the hands flat against the legs.

2 Slowly bend over to the right, sliding the right hand down towards the knee. Your left hand will automatically slide up towards the hip. Allow your head to relax right over.
Hold in your comfortable position for five.

3 Straighten up slowly, pushing down with your left hand to help you. The head comes up only when the body is straight again.

4 Gently relax the head over for a few seconds before repeating on the other side.
Then repeat entire movement again, once each side.

Tummy and Thigh Toner

This movement does exactly what it says it does. It slims and firms the tummy and thighs and helps to strengthen the back.

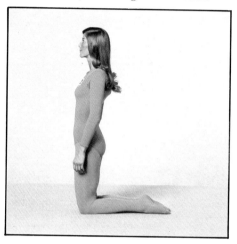

1 Kneel with the back straight, head erect and the arms relaxed at the sides.

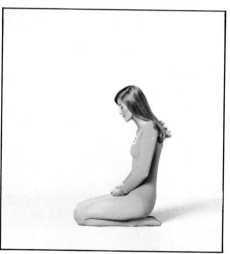

3 When you have executed the movement four times, relax in this position for a few seconds to allow your body to unwind.

You must take care not to bend backwards from the waist. Your body should be in a straight line from the shoulder to the knee as shown in picture 2.

With this movement there is no hold, and it should be executed four times.

Breathing
When kneeling in the upright position, take a deep breath in through the nose – hold the breath as you lean back – straighten up and exhale ready to repeat.

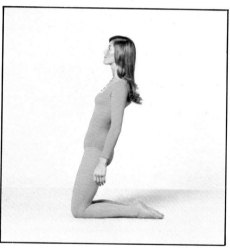

2 Lean back only a few inches – hold for a second or two – and return smoothly to the upright position.

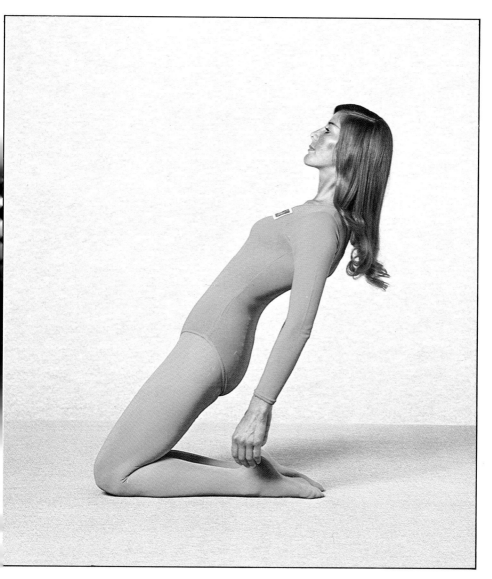

4 With practice it is possible to go further
and further back like this.

The Body Roll

This movement is very effective in eliminating excess flab from around the waist. It also removes stiffness and tension from the neck.

Make sure that you bend forward from the waist and not the hips. To help you do this, push the pelvis forward two or three inches before bending over.

Breathing
Breathe normally and slowly through the nose while executing this movement.

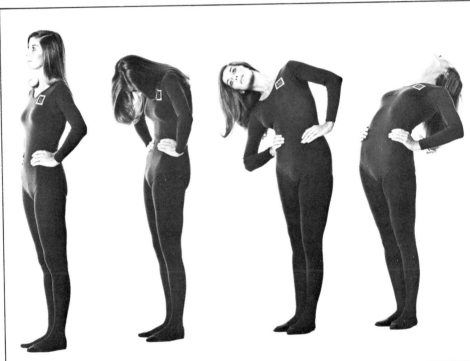

1 Stand with the legs and feet together and grip your waist with your hands.

2 Push the pelvis forward a little and bend over from the waist.

3 Slowly roll the top half of your body around to your right and hold it for a few seconds.

4 Continue on around to the back, allowing the head to go back a little and making sure that the shoulders are back and down. Hold it for a few seconds.

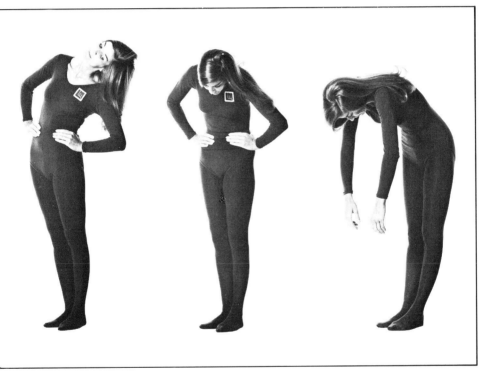

5 Carry on rolling around to your left, and again hold the position for a few seconds.

6 Slowly return to the front.

7 Repeat rotation once more to the right before relaxing like this, then straighten up slowly ready to execute the movement twice round to the left.

Seated Side Bend

This movement gives the sides of the body a really intense stretch.

When you are seated on the floor in this way, your hips are not able to sway in the opposite direction to help you, as often happens with some of the standing side bends. The arms raised with the hands on top of the head also contribute to the stretch.

In order to balance, you must push down really hard with the opposite knee.

As well as stretching the sides of the body and eliminating any excess weight, this movement will strengthen your back and firm the thighs and buttocks. It will also improve your sense of balance and enable you to sit more comfortably in the cross-legged position.

Go over just a few inches at first, as shown in picture 3. You will find that during the hold for five the intensity of the stretch greatly increases, and if you have gone too far it will be a strain to straighten up again.

Make sure that the hands are on top of the head, not the back, as this will push the head forward and cause the top of the spine to curve. Also, make sure that the elbows go straight out to the sides while executing the movement.

Breathing
As you raise the hands to place them on your head, inhale deeply through the nose. Hold the breath as you go over to the side, exhaling during the count. Inhale again as you straighten up and exhale as the head is relaxed forward – ready to repeat.

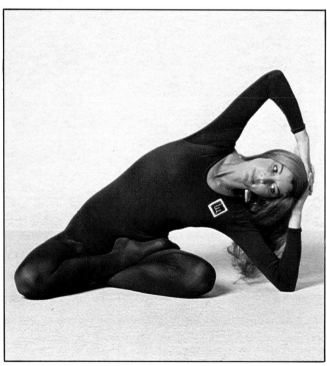

The completed Seated Side Bend
After a lot of practice, you may be able to sit in the Lotus and reach the floor with your elbow like this, but **do not** try it yet.

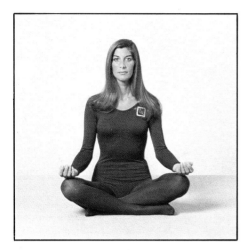

1 Sit with the legs crossed and the hands relaxed on the knees.

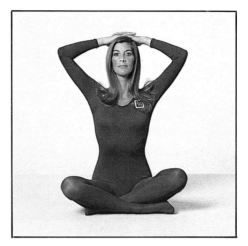

2 Straighten the back, bring the head erect and interlock the fingers, placing the hands on top of the head. Elbows are straight out to the sides.

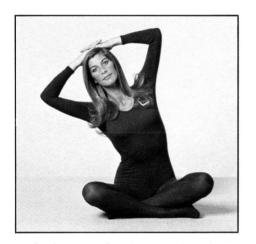

3 Slowly start to bend over to the right, pushing down hard with the left knee to keep the balance.
Hold your position still for a count of five.

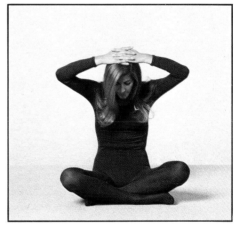

4 Slowly straighten up again and relax like this before repeating on the other side.

The Bow

The Bow really stretches the entire front of the body, from the toes – right up to the head. As you will see from the pictures, the body resembles an archer's bow, and this is how the movement got its name. As well as flexing the back and making it supple and strong, the Bow also greatly strengthens the arms, shoulders and neck, and firms and develops the chest.

If you find that you cannot take the feet as in picture 3, try raising the head and taking first one foot and then the other. As you practise this movement you will find it easier to take the feet as your body and limbs stretch.

Remember to keep the elbows straight all the way through and your knees should stay on the floor for this modified position.

First lie down slowly on to your stomach and relax for a few moments as shown on page 21.

Breathing
Breathe slowly and normally through the nose while executing this movement.

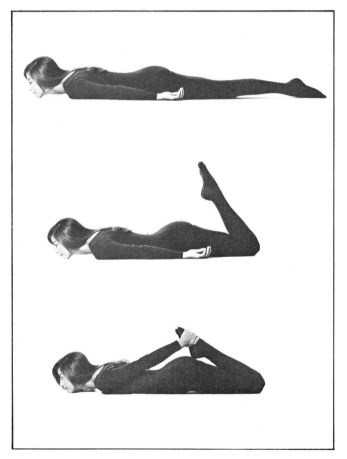

1 Bring the legs and feet together and put the face on to the point of the chin.

2 Start to bend the knees bringing the feet in towards the body.

3 When the feet are as close as they will go, reach back with the hands and try to take the feet.

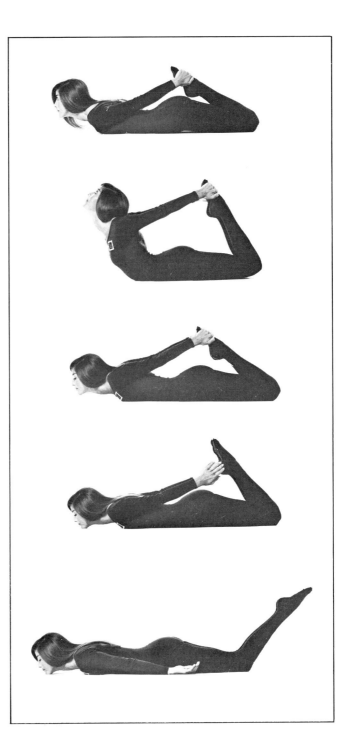

4 Keeping the elbows straight, start to raise the head.

5 Gently push the feet back towards the floor, pulling your shoulders back – then look up and see as much of the ceiling as you can. Hold your position for a count of five.

6 Let your body sink slowly down until your face is resting on the chin again, but do not let go of the feet yet.

7 Take a few seconds and try to regain the muscle control in the legs and feet, so that you can release them without letting them spring out of the hands too much.

8 After lowering your legs slowly to the floor, relax as at the beginning. Wait a few seconds and repeat.

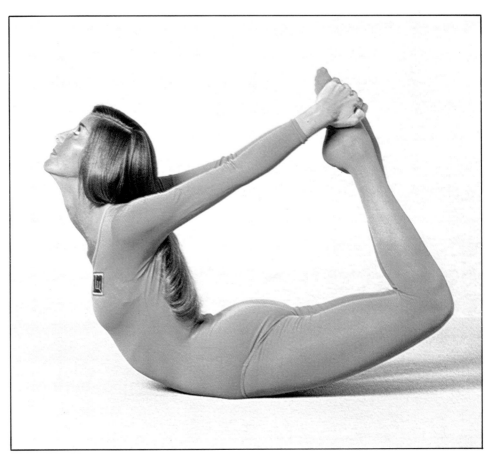

9 After practising the modified position for
a while, you can try this position with
the knees off the floor, causing a more
intense arch in the back. The feet are
pulled up towards the ceiling.

The Squat

This movement not only helps your balance and posture, but also slims and firms the legs and works out stiffness from the knee, toe and ankle joints.

The movement is performed four times and there is no hold.

Breathing

When you are in position with the arms extended, inhale deeply through the nose, exhale as you bend the knees, inhale once more as you straighten up, and exhale in the standing position – ready to repeat.

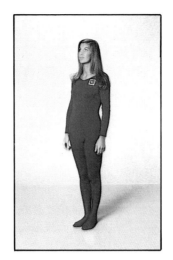

1 Stand with the back straight, head erect and the legs and feet together.

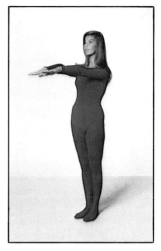

2 Raise the arms so that they are level with the shoulders, turning the palms of the hands towards the floor.

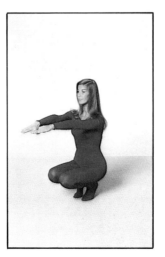

3 Keeping the back as straight as possible, slowly bend the knees and come on to the balls of the feet.

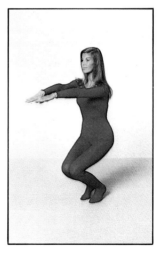

4 Straighten up slowly, ready to repeat.

The Plough

The Plough is the most complete stretch for the back that I have ever come across. It stretches and extends the back from top to bottom.

There are three stages of the Plough, but the second and third stages are extremely difficult and require a lot of practice. They should be considered as advanced postures and not attempted until a great degree of strength and control has been achieved.

We are going to work towards the first position with the feet over the head, shown in picture 7. However, I do not want you to aim to touch the floor with your toes to begin with. Just bring your legs over as far as they will go naturally. With the knees straight, the weight of the legs for the holding count of five will bring them down a little further each time you practise.

Do the movement slowly and with control, and **do not** on any account swing or throw yourself up into the position, as you could do yourself serious harm.

Begin by lying down slowly and relaxing in the Corpse position for a few moments.

Breathing
Take a really deep breath in through the nose before raising the legs – from then on breathe normally and slowly.

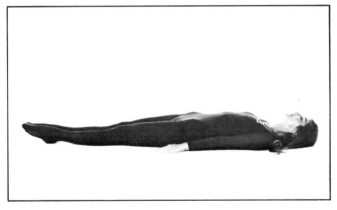

1 Bring the legs and feet together and turn the palms of the hands towards the floor.

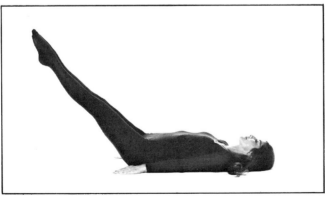

2 Raise your legs, keeping the knees straight and the feet together.

3 Bring the legs over as far as they will go comfortably. Hold the position for five.

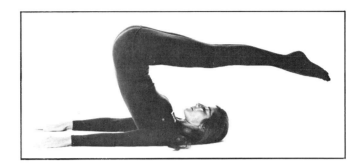

4 Come out of the Plough by bending the knees in towards the chest and tucking the feet in—so that you are in a tight ball.

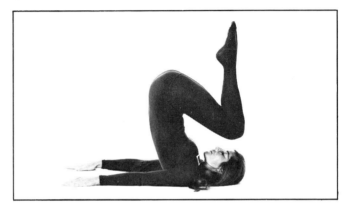

5 Slowly roll out, extending the legs on the way.

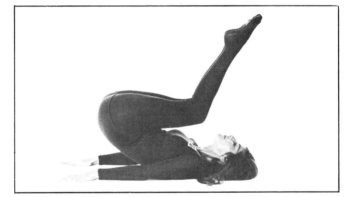

6 Bring the legs smoothly back down to the floor and relax in the Corpse position for a few seconds before repeating.

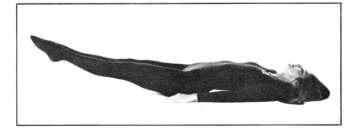

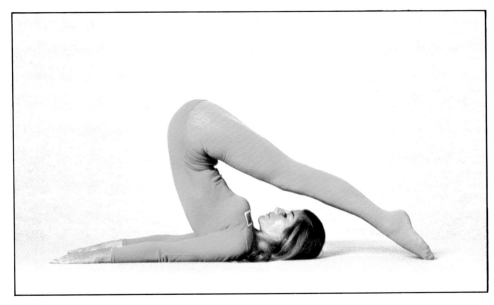

7 This is the completed first position of the
   Plough with the feet touching the floor.

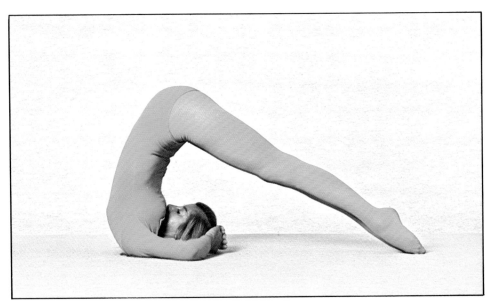

8 Completed second position, with the legs
  extended further away from the head by
  pushing down on the head with the hands.

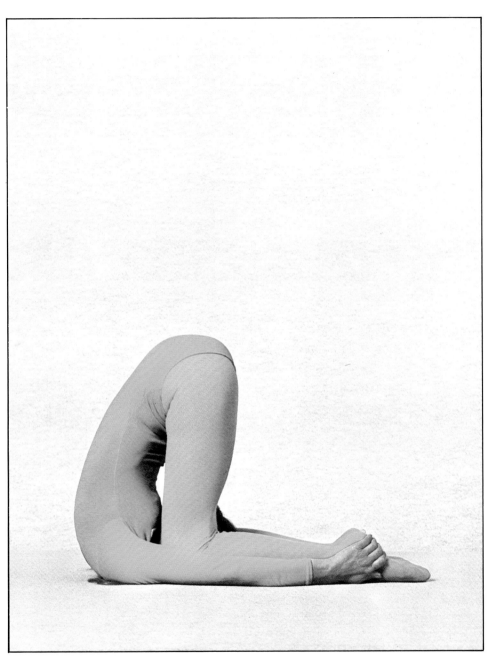

9 Completed third position of the Plough,
with the knees brought in beside the ears.

The Locust

This movement may look deceptively easy, but it actually requires a lot of strength to raise the legs in this manner. It is a marvellously invigorating movement to do, and one that will tighten and firm the buttock and leg muscles as well as strengthening the back.

It is also one of the few Yoga movements that is partially designed to exercize the heart, causing it to beat faster during the hold. Do not become alarmed when this happens, but do make sure that you relax as shown in picture 1 for at least thirty seconds after performing the movement, so that the heart beat can return to normal.

Although you are lying on your stomach, you must take a really deep breath before raising the legs, as once in position you are forced to hold the breath.

Remember to keep the chin on the floor, and raise only a few inches at first. Also, the legs and feet must be together with the knees absolutely straight.

WARNING
This movement should not be attempted by anyone suffering from high blood pressure or any other heart condition.

Breathing
Take a deep breath in through the nose before raising the legs – hold it for the count – exhale slowly as the legs are lowered.

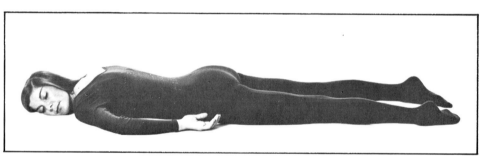

1 Lie down slowly and relax for a few moments by putting the face on the cheek, allowing the heels to fall right open, and bending the elbows slightly to relax the shoulders, arms and fingers.

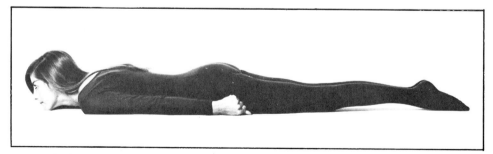

2 Bring the legs and feet together and put the face on to the point of the chin. Straighten the elbows and make fists of the hands with the thumbs towards the floor.

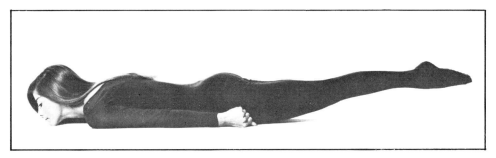

3 Take a deep breath, push down hard with the fists, and raise the legs, keeping the knees straight and the feet together.
Hold your position for five.

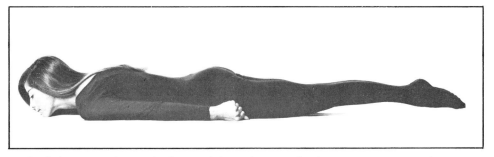

4 Slowly lower your legs to the floor and then relax completely again as in picture 1 for at least thirty seconds before repeating the movement a second time.

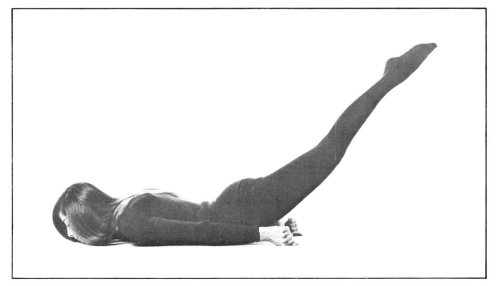

5 After much practice, it is possible to achieve a higher raise – like this.

Front Push-up

This movement improves the complexion by allowing blood to flow freely into the face. It strengthens the wrists, arms, shoulders and toes and also gently stretches the backs of the legs.

The holding count for this position is five, but until your arms strengthen, you may find that they are shaking a little during the count. If this is so, then reduce the holding count to three. You can gradually increase it as your arms strengthen with practice.

Breathing
When in position on the hands and knees, take a deep breath in through the nose – push up and then continue to breathe slowly and normally.

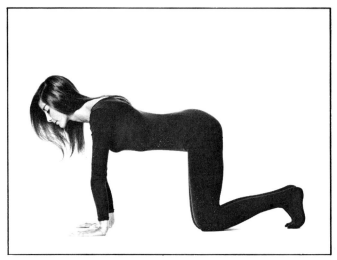

1 Come on to the hands and knees and try to place your hands directly underneath your shoulders. Tuck the toes under so that you are resting on the balls of the feet.

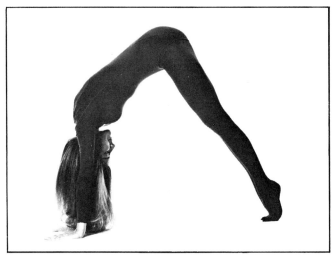

2 Push up, straightening the elbows and the knees, and allow the head to relax completely – just let it hang. Hold your position for a count of five.

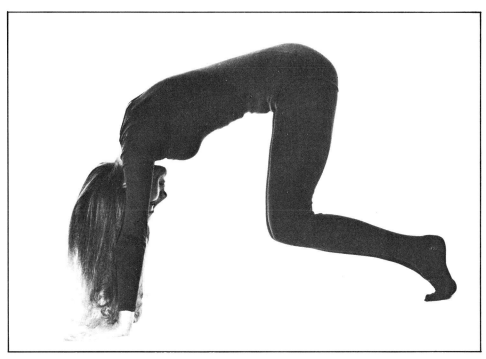

3 Slowly lower the knees and return to your starting position. (Pressing the knees together as you lower will help you to come down slowly and smoothly.)
The head can stay relaxed forward while you wait a few seconds before repeating.

4 After executing the movement twice, relax in this position to allow the body to unwind.

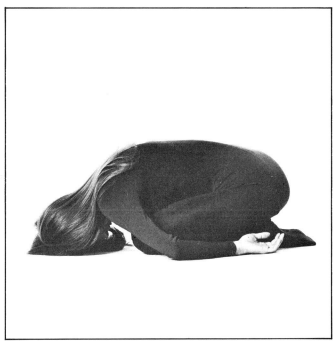

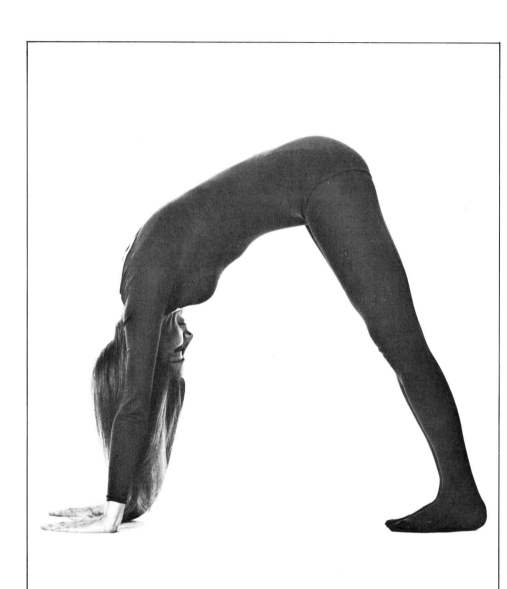

5 With this variation there is no hold.
  Instead, the heels are gently lowered
  towards the floor three times, increasing
  the stretch at the backs of the legs.

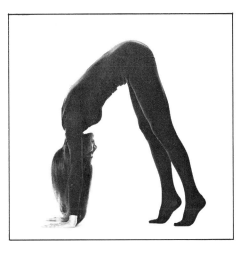

6 A more advanced variation is to take little steps in towards the hands – pausing three or four times to lower the heels.

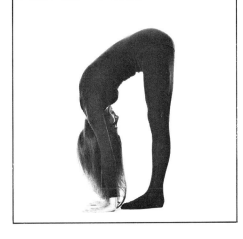

7 Until eventually the feet are almost touching the hands.

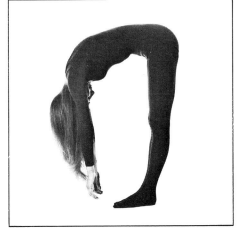

8 It is then possible to transfer the weight from the arms on to the legs – and straighten up slowly.
   This variation requires a lot of strength and control, so do not try it yet.

Complete Breath – Standing

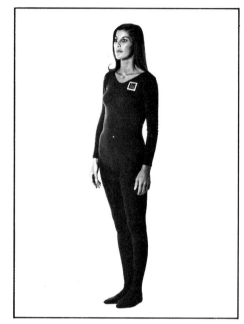

By raising and lowering the arms as you inhale and exhale, you are helping the lungs to function efficiently, and taking in as much oxygen as you can with each breath. This intake of oxygen will serve to recharge your entire organism.

The practice of the Complete Breath will have a tremendously revitalizing effect, which will be felt immediately. Also, it will greatly improve your breathing generally.

1 Stand with the back straight, head erect and the legs and feet together.

Complete Breath – Lying

The benefits of this movement are exactly the same as for the Standing Complete Breath, but it is important for you to know how to execute it both standing and lying down.

1 Lie on the floor with the legs and feet together.

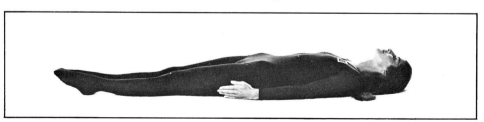

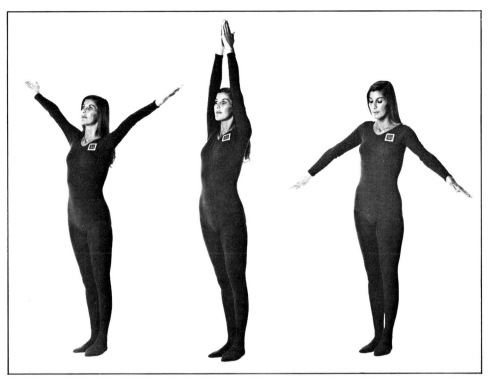

2 Inhale deeply, and at the same time bring the arms slowly up with the palms uppermost.

3 Until the hands meet above the head.

4 Exhale slowly as you lower the arms back down to your sides – ready to repeat immediately. Execute the movement eight times in all.

2 Inhale deeply and at the same time raise the arms until the hands meet above, the head.
Then exhale lowering the arms slowly back to your sides – ready to repeat immediately.

Execute the movement eight times in all.

Note
The hands should brush the floor as the arms are raised and lowered.

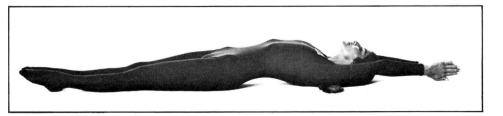

The Coil

This movement really increases strength and mobility in the neck and stretches the very top of the spine. It also firms and trims the buttocks.

Make sure that the elbows go down towards the floor as in picture 4, and spend a few moments relaxing in the Corpse before you begin.

Breathing
When in position with the hands looped around the knees, take a deep breath in through the nose – pull on the knees and exhale as you bring the head up. Remain without breath for the count. Inhale as you lower the head to the floor, and exhale when you are flat, ready to repeat.

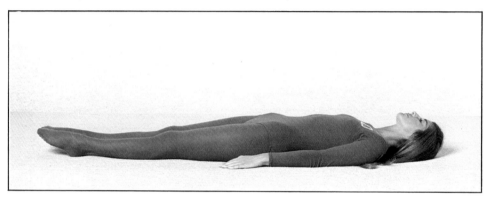

1 Lie with the legs and feet together and the palms of the hands towards the floor.

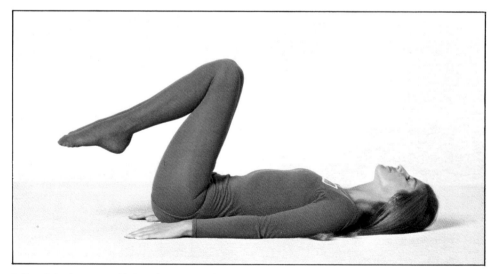

2 Bend the knees and bring them in as close to the chest as you can.

3 Interlock the fingers and loop the hands over the knees.

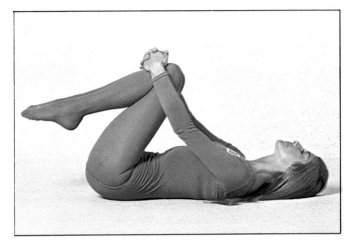

4 Pull on the knees with the hands and raise your head towards the knees. Hold the position for five.

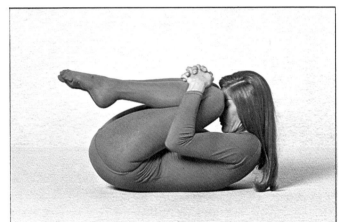

5 Lower the head to the floor and relax like this for a few seconds before repeating.

After executing the movement twice, undo the fingers and bring the arms back down to the sides, extend the legs and relax in the Corpse for a few moments to allow the body to unwind.

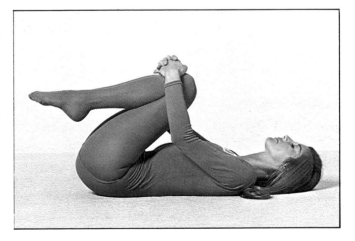

Standing Leg Grip

This movement stretches the back and the muscles and ligaments in the legs. It also stretches the neck and allows fresh blood to flow into the head and face, refreshing them.

It is important that you do not attempt to grip the legs any lower down than where the hands are hanging relaxed, and that the elbows go out to the sides during the stretch.

Breathing

When in position with the elbows straight, take a deep breath in through the nose – hold it as you pull on the legs, bringing the head in, and for the count. Exhale after you have straightened the elbows and raised the head slightly. Breathe normally for a few seconds before repeating.

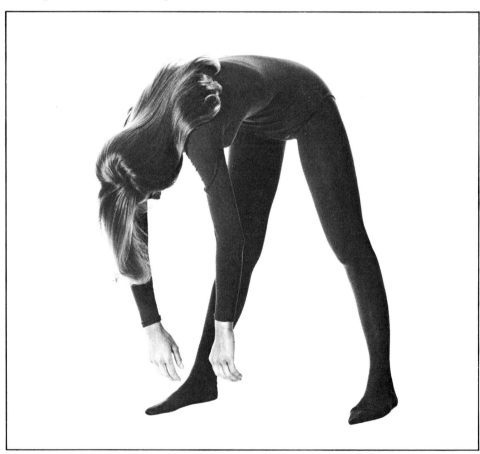

1 Stand with the legs and feet about twenty inches apart and relax forward as for the Refresher* movement, allowing the head, hands and arms to hang completely.

*See *Wake up to Yoga* p. 16

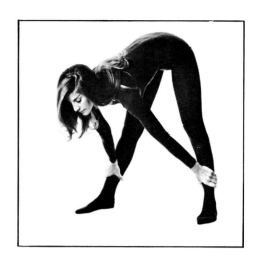

2 Grip the legs and raise the head slightly, keeping the elbows straight.

3 Pull on the legs, letting the elbows go out to the side and bring the head in as far as you can.
Hold the position for five.

4 Let the elbows straighten slowly and bring the head up a little. Relax for a few moments before repeating.

After you have executed the movement twice, relax once more in the Refresher as picture 1, and straighten up slowly, bringing the head up last.

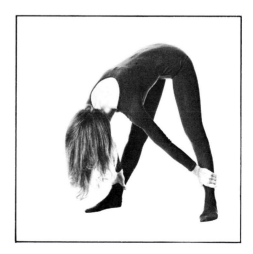

Lotus Instruction

Although it is perfectly all right to do the seated movements in a simple cross-legged position, once you can sit comfortably in a half or full Lotus, your position becomes much more stable. Do not, however, become impatient if it takes a while to get into the Lotus. Remember that your limbs have to stretch very gently until they become used to the position.

The first requisite of the Lotus is to be able to get the knees down on to the floor.

If you practise the following a few times each day, you will gradually find your knees going down. Also, the practice of movements such as the Alternate Leg Pull, the Thigh Stretch, the Seated Side Bend and the Full Twist will help you towards this.

Note
The Leg Pull, Thigh Stretch and Full Twist movements referred to are contained in the book *Wake up to Yoga*.

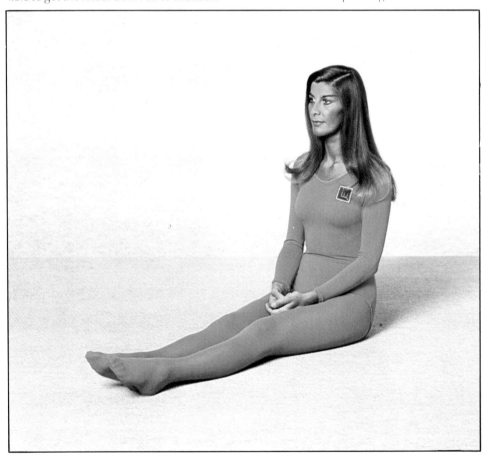

1 Sit on the floor with both legs stretched out in front of you.

2 Bend the right knee and bring the foot over to rest on the left thigh.

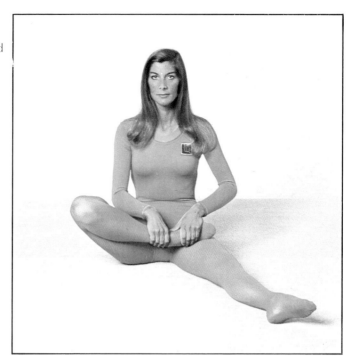

3 Now, simply rest the right wrist on the knee completely relaxing the arm. The weight of the arm and hand will gently push the knee towards the floor.
Hold the position until it becomes uncomfortable, then change legs.

Eventually, when one knee rests comfortably on the floor, you can try the Half Lotus position shown on page 52.

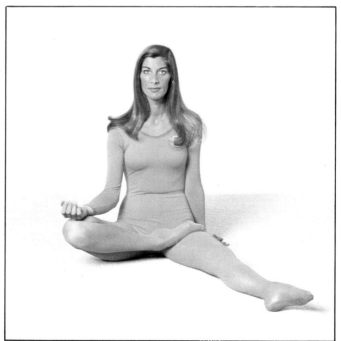

The Half Lotus

1 Bend the knee and bring the sole of the foot in along the inside of the other thigh.

2 Bring the other foot over to rest on the thigh.

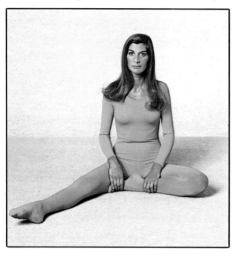 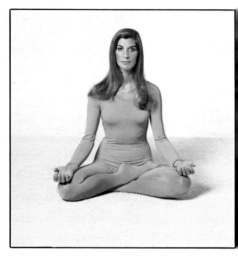

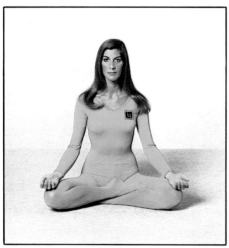 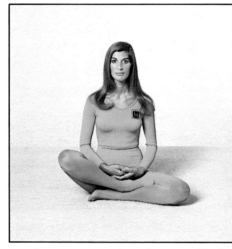

3 Alternatively, if it is more comfortable, it can be placed in the cleft between the thigh and the calf.

4 It does not matter if your knee is still high up like this. With regular practice it will go down.
Remain in the position only as long as it is comfortable, then extend the legs carefully. Massage the knees if they feel a little stiff and relax all the leg and feet muscles for a few moments.

The Full Lotus

The Full Lotus position is achieved as follows:

1 Bend one knee and place the foot on the opposite thigh.

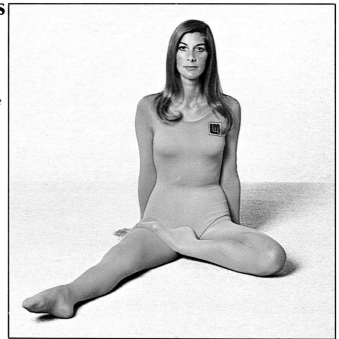

2 Then do the same with the other leg.

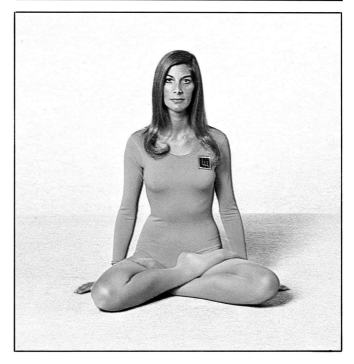

Eye Rotations

This movement exercizes the eye muscles, eliminating strain and tension.

Do not allow the head to move, and hold each position of the eyes for a second or two.

Breathing
Breathe normally and slowly through the nose while executing this movement.

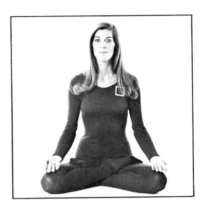

1 Sit in a comfortable position with the back straight and the head erect.

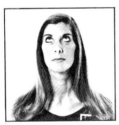

2 Without moving the head, look up as far as you can.

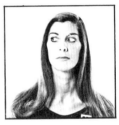

3 Roll the eyes as far round to the right as you can.

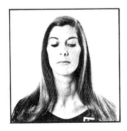

4 Roll the eyes down and look as low as you can without moving the head.

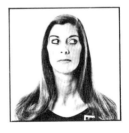

5 Continue round to your extreme left. Repeat rotation once more and then execute twice in opposite direction before closing the eyes and relaxing for a few moments.

Ante- and Post-Natal Section

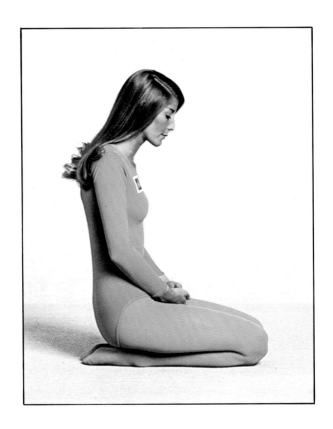

Caution
Before commencing with any of the
following movements you must obtain the
full permission of your doctor.

Abdominal Deep Breathing

The ability to relax and breathe deeply will be of great assistance to you when you come actually to give birth. The practice of this movement will help you to achieve both. You can also practise the Abdominal Breathing exercize on page 22.

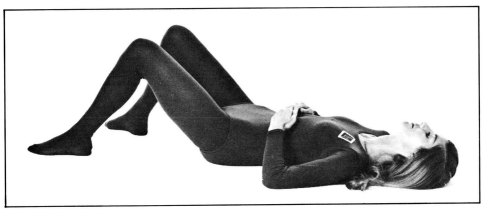

1 Lie flat on your back with the knees bent and the feet apart.
Check that you are breathing correctly by placing the hands on the abdomen so that you can feel the rise and fall as you breathe in and out.

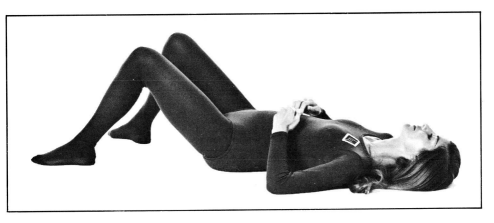

2 Inhale slowly through the nose, allowing the abdomen to expand, then the diaphragm and the chest.
Hold the breath for a few seconds and then exhale gently and slowly, allowing the breath to creep out as you feel the chest, diaphragm and abdomen sink down.

You should practise this deep breathing every day if possible for five to ten minutes. After a while, try to inhale and hold the breath for a few seconds before exhaling, and gradually increase the period of breath retention.

57

Thigh Stretch Variation

This movement loosens the knee and hip joints and stretches the legs, especially the very top of the inside thigh. It also prepares the body for childbirth by stretching the pelvic floor.

Take care not to jerk as you push the knees down, and do not expect a great deal of movement to begin with. This area of the leg is unused to being stretched in this way, so be patient with yourself.

Breathing

When in position as picture 3 inhale deeply through the nose. Exhale as you push the knees down with the elbows, and retain your position without breath. Inhale again as you allow the knees to come up, and exhale as you relax ready to repeat.

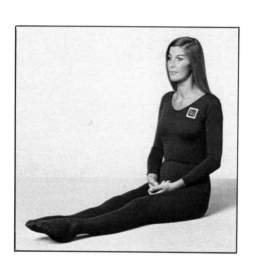

1 Sit on the floor with the legs stretched out in front of you.

2 Bend the knees, and gripping the ankles pull the feet in towards you.

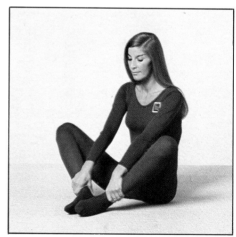

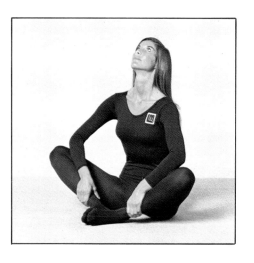

3 Straighten the back as much as you can, raise the chin and rest the elbows on the knees.

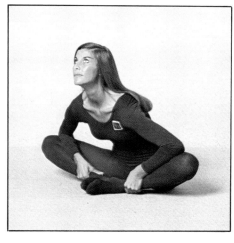

4 Still gripping the ankles, gently push the knees down towards the floor and bear forwards with the trunk.
Stop as soon as you become aware of the stretch on the inside of the upper thigh, and hold your position still for a count of five.

5 Allow the knees to come up, and relax for a few seconds before repeating.

Execute the movement four times in all before extending the legs straight out in front of you and relaxing all the leg and feet muscles.

The Cat

The Cat is a very valuable ante-natal movement and can be practised throughout your entire pregnancy. It will retain strength and suppleness in the spine without putting a strain on the abdominal region.

You may find that your elbows have a tendency to bend during the movement – don't let them – they should remain absolutely straight all the time.

Execute the movement very slowly and smoothly, and take care to spend a few moments at the end relaxing as shown in picture 6.

Breathing
Breathe normally and slowly through the nose while executing the movement.

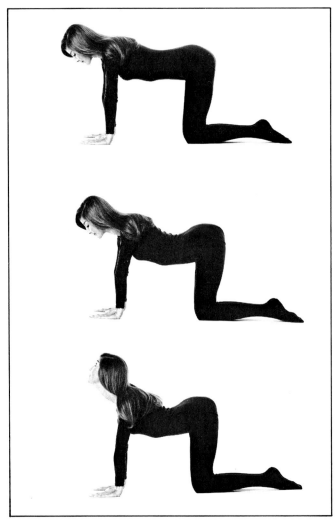

1 Come on to the hands and knees, placing the hands directly underneath the shoulders.

2 Slowly let the back sink down, pushing the bottom right up and out.

3 Raise the face and see as much of the ceiling as you can.
Hold the position for a count of five.

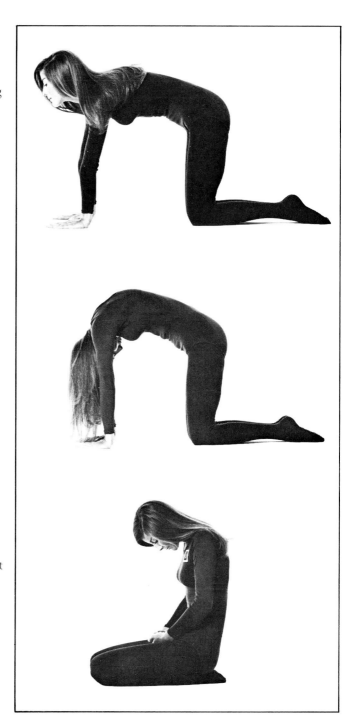

4 Now slowly reverse the
   position by arching the
   back and gently pushing
   the pelvis forward.

5 Try to get the chin right
   down on to the chest.
   Hold your position for a
   count of five and
   immediately repeat
   entire movement.

6 When you have
   executed the movement
   twice, relax by sitting
   back on to the heels
   and remaining in this
   position for a few
   moments. Then repeat
   twice more.

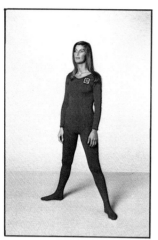

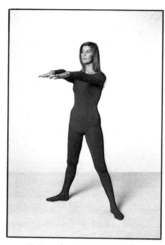

The Squat Variation

This is a variation of the movement on page 33, but it is executed with the legs apart, pressing the knees open as much as possible as you bend. Also, with this variation, do not rise up on to the balls of the feet.

Keep the head erect and the back as straight as you can as you bend the knees.

1 Stand with the legs about twenty inches apart and the toes pointing out to the corners.

2 Bring the arms straight up in front of you with the palms of the hands towards the floor, fingers straight.

Breathing
When in position as picture 2, inhale deeply through the nose, exhale as you bend the knees, inhale once more as you straighten up, and exhale in the starting position ready to repeat.

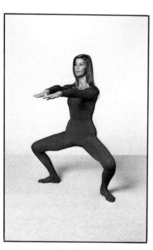

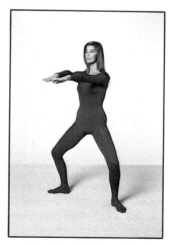

3 Keeping the back straight and the head erect, bend the knees as far as is comfortable.

4 Slowly straighten up without jerking, and remain in position ready to repeat.
Execute down–up movement four times.

Other Recommended Movements

Other movements that you can practise
from this book are:
Standing Slide Bend (page 23)
Complete Breath – Standing (page 44)
Complete Breath – Lying (page 44)
Eye Rotations (page 54)

The following movements can be practised
from the book *Wake up to Yoga*:
The Corpse (deep relaxation)
Tension Release – basic movement only
The Fish – as instructed
Balance Posture – as instructed
Scissors – down only to the knee
Triangle – down only to the knee
Alternate Nostril Breathing – gradually
increasing count to six

The following are seated movements and
can be executed either in the cross-legged
position or kneeling and sitting back on
the heels, or, if more comfortable in the
later stages of pregnancy, sitting on
a chair.
Finger Pulls – execute with breathing
instructions given in index
Neck Roll – as instructed
Jaw Lift – as instructed
Scalp Tugs – as instructed
Foot Rotations – as instructed
Elbow Snaps – as instructed
The Lion – as instructed or as on page 75 of
this book

Post-Natal

The period immediately after your baby is born is crucial, and you must get the muscles working as soon as you can if you are to avoid sagging.

The following movements can be done sitting or lying in bed as soon as the day after your baby is born, and although they are subtle they are extremely effective.

Before you commence with these or any of the other recommended post-natal movements, **you must obtain the full permission of your doctor.**

Vaginal and Abdominal Contractions

These contractions are extremely valuable and can be commenced as soon after the birth as your doctor permits. They will help to tighten up the pelvic floor, preventing the possibility of prolapse of the uterus and the vagina later on in life.

Vaginal Contractions

Lie on your back in bed and relax. Contract the vagina and feel the same sort of sensation as when you are preventing the bladder from working.
Hold for a few seconds, relax and repeat.
Execute the contracting movement ten times in all and repeat twice a day.

Abdominal Contractions

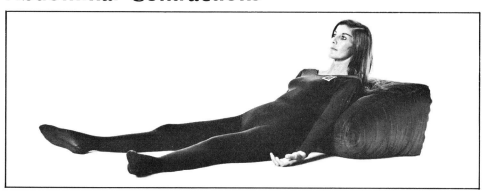

1 Sit or lie in bed with the legs, feet, arms and hands completely relaxed.

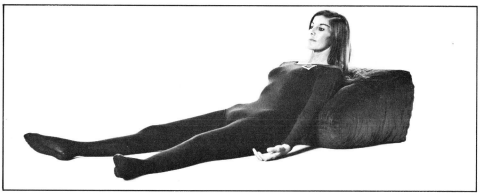

2 Pull the abdomen in and up as much as possible, and hold it for a slow count of five.
   Relax the muscles, wait a few seconds and repeat.
   Perform the contraction movement six times and try to repeat at least twice a day.
   With practice, gradually increase the holding count of ten.

Alternate Leg Raise

This movement, like the two previous ones, can be done lying in bed.

Raise the right leg with the knee straight just a few inches. Hold for a count of five.

Lower the leg slowly, keeping the knee straight. Repeat with the left leg.

Repeat twice more with each leg before relaxing. With practice you can gradually increase the holding period to ten, and execute the movement twice a day if possible.

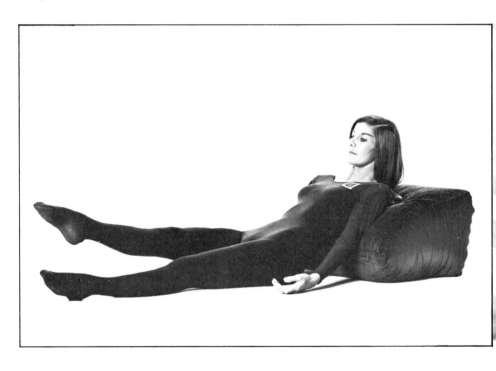

Additional Tips

Once you are out of bed, try to walk in a
very erect fashion with the shoulders back
and the head up. Although you may feel a
little silly at first, imitate a model's walk,
pushing the pelvis forward and pinching the
buttocks in. Even if you do this for just a few
minutes each day, you will find that it is of
great help and will accelerate the return of
your figure.

Also, you can start gently to practise other
movements both from this book and from
Wake up to Yoga, but exactly WHEN to
commence certain movements depends
entirely on the condition of the individual.
Each case is different, so once again I would
urge you always to consult your doctor first.

Sit Up – Lie Down

This movement, as the name suggests, entails sitting up and lying down, but without the use of your hands – making all your muscles work.

You should not attempt it until you are out of bed, and only then with the full approval of your doctor.

Try to do the movement in extreme slow motion, without jerking. It will strengthen and tighten the abdominal muscles, the bottom and the thighs, and strengthen the back, the shoulders, the arms and the neck.

If you find it really impossible to sit up without using your hands, then to begin with hook your toes underneath something heavy, like an armchair or settee, but the sooner you can do the movement unaided the better.

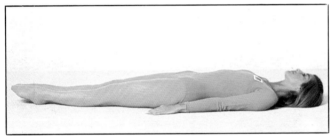

1 Lie down slowly flat on your back, with the legs and feet together and arms by your side.

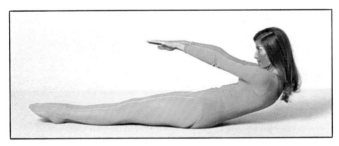

2 Really make a big effort as you reach forward with the arms.

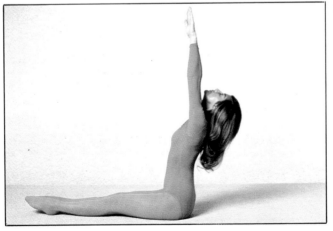

3 Try to sit straight up with your arms above your head.

4 Bring your hands down on to your legs and lower your chin to your chest.

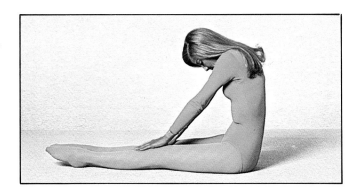

5 Start to roll slowly back down the spine, keeping the elbows straight and the shoulders hunched and pushing down hard with the toes.

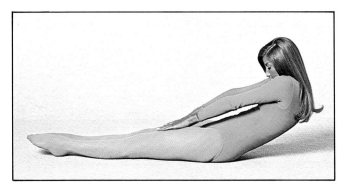

6 Carry on rolling slowly, and after the back has touched the floor let the head go back, and go into the Corpse position by allowing the toes to fall open and relaxing the hands.
Stay like this for a few seconds and repeat. You should execute the sitting up and lying down movement four times in all, and if possible repeat it twice a day.

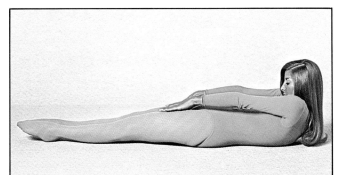

Progressions and Variations of Movements covered in 'Wake up to Yoga'

The following are advanced variations and progressions of movements taught in the book *Wake up to Yoga*. Please do not attempt them until you have practised and mastered the basic movements.

The Cobra

1 When you can com-
fortably hold the full
Cobra position with the
elbows straight, you can
continue with this
advanced variation.

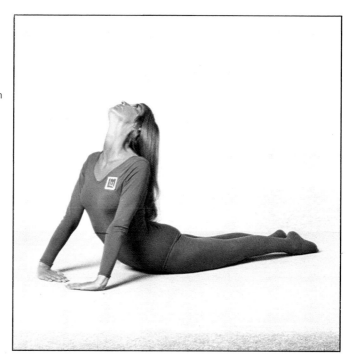

2 Slowly bend the right
elbow, keeping the left
straight, and slowly turn
the head to the left to see
the back of the left heel.
Hold your position for a
count of five, turn the
head back slowly and
straighten the right
elbow, going once more
into the full Cobra with
the shoulders back and
down and the head right
back.
Repeat on the other
side, and come out of
the position in the usual
way, closing the eyes if
you wish.

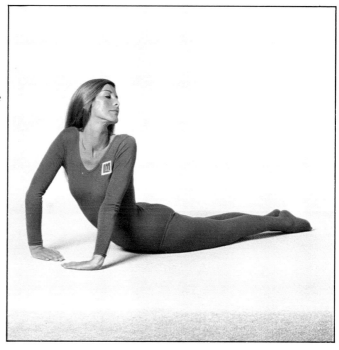

Leg Pulls

When you can comfortably take hold of the
ankles and have been practising for a while,
you can try this variation, but you must
incorporate the correct breathing as
instructed in *Wake up to Yoga* (page 93).

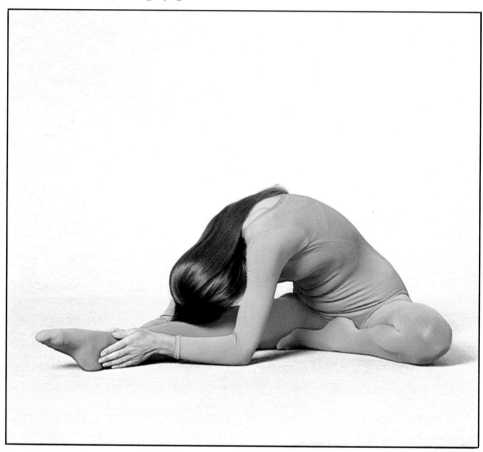

The elbows go down towards the floor,
intensifying the stretch at the back of the
leg and the base of the back.

Backward Bend

When you are quite comfortable in the basic Backward Bend position, you can try this variation.

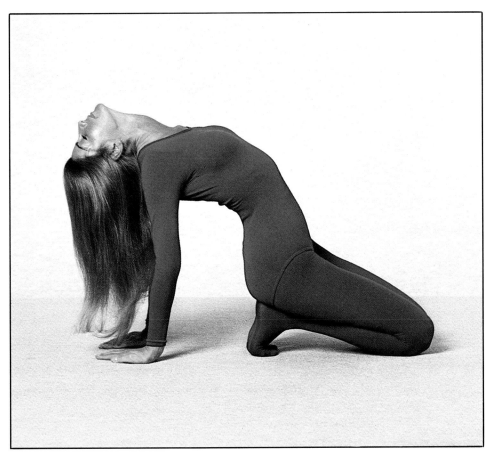

The toes are tucked under and your weight is resting on the balls of the feet. In this position the arch in the back is more intense.

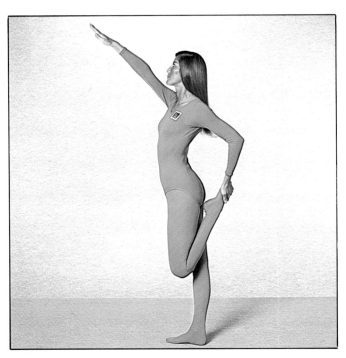

Balance Posture

1 When you have mastered this basic upright position and are able to maintain it securely for quite a few seconds, continue on as follows.

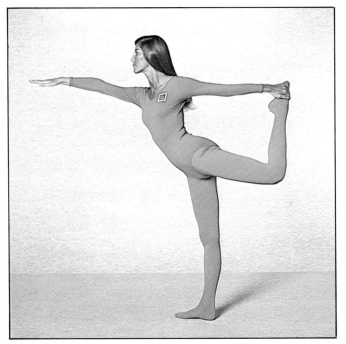

2 Bring the arm down slowly until it is parallel with the floor and rock forwards a little from the hips. Then extend the raised leg a little keeping hold of the foot. Maintain the position for a few seconds, then rock back carefully to picture 1 and come out of the position in the normal way.

Lion Variation

This is an alternative way of executing the Lion movement.

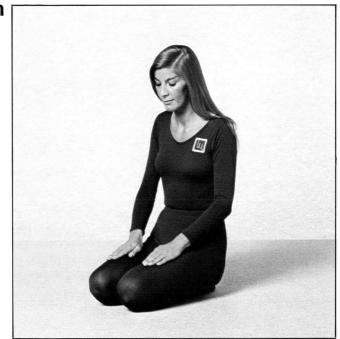

1 The Lion kneeling

2 The Lion completed

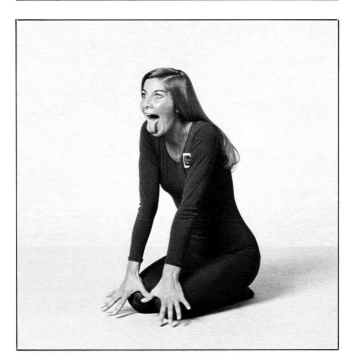

Note

The following are progressive breathing instructions that can be used with the appropriate movements and variations of movements covered in *Wake up to Yoga*.

The Twist

When in position, take a deep breath in through the nose – hold the breath as you twist round and for the count – twist back and exhale, relaxing for a few seconds before repeating.

Slow Motion Firming

As you bend the knees in toward the chest, inhale deeply through the nose. Hold the breath as you extend the legs and exhale as the legs are lowered to the floor. Inhale as you reach forward and sit up, hold the breath while taking the legs and pulling the body forward, and exhale as the head relaxes over. Inhale gently as you roll back down the spine, exhaling when you are flat again, ready to repeat.

Practice Sessions

These routines for twenty and thirty minutes are examples of the way various movements can be put together to form practice sessions. It is fine for you to follow them, but please remember that I have constructed these routines purely as examples, and you can interchange the movements as you wish both from this book and from *Wake up to Yoga*. The only requisite is that you maintain a balance by doing movements that will get to as much of the body as possible.

Do not try to cram too many movements into any one session. To rush the movements would be to ruin your chances of receiving the full benefits of Yoga. The slower you do the movements the better, and if this means that you must eliminate one or more movements from your session, then do so. Never feel tempted to speed up in order to get all the movements in.

Note

Whatever movements you choose for your session, **you must always** spend at least a few minutes relaxing completely in the Corpse position both at the beginning and at the end of the session (see page 20).

Sessions for 20 minutes

1 CORPSE

COMPLETE BREATH–STANDING

BODY ROLL

BOW

PLOUGH

CORPSE

2 CORPSE

STANDING SLIDE BEND

FRONT PUSH-UP

BOW

LOCUST

CORPSE

Sessions for 30 minutes

1 CORPSE

COMPLETE BREATH–STANDING

BODY ROLL

TUMMY AND THIGH TONER

BOW

THE COIL

CORPSE

2 CORPSE

COMPLETE BREATH–LYING

STANDING LEG GRIP

SQUAT

SEATED SIDE BEND

LOCUST

CORPSE

Index of Movements and Postures

38–9 The Locust
To greatly strengthen the back, and to slim and firm the legs, thighs, hips and buttocks.

40–3 Front Push-up
To improve the complexion by inverting the head, increasing the blood flow to the head and face.
To stretch the back and the backs of the legs.
To greatly strengthen the shoulders, arms and wrists.

44–5 Complete Breath – Standing
To enable the lungs to function efficiently and improve your breathing generally.
To revitalize yourself and to recharge your entire organism.

44–5 Complete Breath – Lying
This movement has all the benefits of the Complete Breath – Standing, and is an alternative way of executing the movement.

46–7 The Coil
To stretch the very top of the spine.
To increase strength and mobility in the neck.
To trim and firm the buttocks and thighs.

48–9 Standing Leg Grip
To stretch and strengthen the back and the muscles and ligaments in the legs.
To strengthen the shoulders, arms and neck.
To refresh the head and face and improve the complexion by inverting the head, increasing the blood flow to the head and face.
To improve blood circulation generally throughout the body.

50–3 Lotus Instruction
To help you to achieve the Half Lotus and eventually, the Full Lotus positions comfortably.

54 Eye Rotations
To exercize the eye muscles, eliminating strain and tension from the eyes.

Ante- and Post-Natal Section

(ANTE-NATAL)

57 Abdominal Deep Breathing
To learn the art of relaxation and deep breathing at the same time.
To learn breath retention.

58–9 Thigh Stretch Variation
To stretch the pelvic floor in preparation for childbirth.
To loosen the knee and hip joints and stretch the legs, especially the very top of the inside thigh.
To improve your breathing generally.

60–1 The Cat
A highly valuable ante-natal movement as it will promote a great degree of suppleness and strength in the back without putting a strain on the abdomen.
It will also trim and firm the buttocks, hips and thighs, and strengthen the neck, shoulders, arms and wrists.

62 **The Squat Variation**

To promote good posture during pregnancy.

To strengthen the back and the leg muscles, and to stretch the inside of the upper thigh.

To improve your breathing generally.

(POST-NATAL)

65 **Vaginal Contractions**

To help tighten up the pelvic floor, preventing the possibility of prolapse of the uterus and the vagina later on in life.

65 **Abdominal Contractions**

To firm and flatten the abdomen, and to regain muscle tone in that area.

66 **Alternate Leg Raise**

To slim and firm the legs, thighs and tummy.

68–9 **Sit Up – Lie Down**

To strengthen and firm the abdominal muscles.

To slim and firm the legs, thighs, bottom, hips and waist.

To strengthen the back, shoulders, arms and neck.

Progressions and Variations of Movements

71 **The Cobra**

To increase the strength in the shoulders, arms and neck.

72 **Leg Pulls**

To intensify the stretch at the back of the leg and the base of the back.

73 **Backward Bend**

To create a more intense arch in the back and to strengthen and work out stiffness from the toes.

74 **Balance Posture**

To increase your powers of concentration and balance.

To greatly increase muscle control throughout the entire body.

75 **Lion Variation**

An alternative way of executing the Lion movement.